Blueberries Growing Guide for Beginners

Choosing the Right Varieties of Blueberries

By

Darian Ewan

Copyright@2023

Table of Contents

CHAPTER 1

Introduction

1.1 Overview of Blueberries

The blueberry, a delightful and nutritious fruit, belongs to the genus Vaccinium and encompasses various species native to North America, Europe, and Asia. Primarily known for their sweet-tart flavor profile and vibrant blue hue, blueberries have gained immense popularity as a versatile ingredient in culinary endeavors, a health-conscious snack, and an attractive addition to gardens and landscapes.

Cultural and Culinary Significance:
Blueberries boast a rich cultural history, deeply rooted in indigenous communities where they held significance as a staple food and medicinal resource. Their utilization extended beyond sustenance; blueberries found their way into traditional

ceremonies and folklore, symbolizing health, renewal, and harmony with nature.

The versatility of blueberries in culinary applications is remarkable. From pies to jams, smoothies to salads, their tangy sweetness adds a delightful dimension to an array of dishes. Their antioxidants and nutritional value have also made them a celebrated superfood in modern diets, contributing to improved health and well-being.

Botanical Insights: Blueberries belong to the Ericaceae family, and their taxonomy encompasses several species, including Vaccinium corymbosum (highbush), Vaccinium angustifolium (lowbush), and Vaccinium ashei (rabbiteye). These species vary in size, flavor, and preferred growing conditions.

Their growth habit, characterized by woody perennial shrubs, showcases delicate, bell-shaped flowers in spring, which transform into clusters of berries ranging in size from small marbles to larger varieties. Blueberries often exhibit a range of colors from deep blue to purple-black, each variant offering its unique taste profile and culinary applications.

Health and Nutritional Benefits: Blueberries stand out not only for their exquisite taste but also for their health benefits. Packed with antioxidants, vitamins C and K, manganese, and dietary fiber, these berries are celebrated for their potential to promote heart health, improve cognitive function, and aid in managing oxidative stress. Research continues to unveil their role in reducing the risk of chronic diseases and supporting overall wellness.

Cultivation and Global Presence: The cultivation of blueberries has expanded globally, with regions like North America, South America, Europe, and Oceania emerging as significant producers. Understanding the optimal conditions for growth—such as acidic soil, adequate sunlight, and proper irrigation—is pivotal for successful cultivation.

Blueberries thrive in diverse environments, from small-scale home gardens to expansive commercial farms, contributing significantly to agricultural economies worldwide. Growers employ various cultivation techniques and harvesting methods to ensure the quality and yield of these prized fruits.

1.2 Benefits of Growing Blueberries

The decision to grow blueberries extends far beyond the delight of harvesting fresh fruit. Cultivating these berries brings forth a multitude of benefits that span environmental, health, economic, and even aesthetic realms. Here's a detailed exploration of the benefits:

1. Health and Nutrition:

- **Nutrient-Rich Fruit:** Blueberries are a nutritional powerhouse, packed with antioxidants, vitamins

C and K, fiber, and various other essential nutrients. Growing your own ensures access to fresh, pesticide-free berries rich in health-boosting properties.

- **Promotes Healthy Eating:** Cultivating blueberries encourages a diet rich in fruits, fostering a habit of consuming nutrient-dense, whole foods.

2. Economic Value:

- **Personal Savings:** Growing blueberries at home reduces grocery expenses, providing a cost-effective source of high-quality, organic fruit.

- **Potential Income:** For larger-scale cultivation, blueberry farming can serve as a lucrative endeavor, contributing to agricultural revenue in local markets.

3. Environmental Benefits:

- **Biodiversity Support:** Blueberry bushes attract pollinators such as bees and butterflies, contributing to local biodiversity and ecosystem health.

- **Sustainable Cultivation:** Employing eco-friendly practices in blueberry cultivation, such as natural pest control and organic fertilizers, supports sustainable agriculture.

4. Aesthetic Appeal:

- **Garden Enhancement:** Blueberry bushes offer ornamental value with their delicate flowers in spring, colorful foliage in autumn, and the allure of the ripening berries throughout the summer.

5. Educational Value:

- **Learning Experience:** Growing blueberries provides an educational opportunity for children and adults alike to understand plant growth cycles, soil health, and the importance of sustainable agriculture.

6. Community and Social Aspects:

- **Sharing and Bonding:** A surplus of blueberries can be shared with neighbors, fostering community connections and a sense of generosity.

- **Engagement and Events:** Blueberry picking events or community gardening projects centered around blueberry cultivation can bring people together, promoting social interaction and cooperation.

7. Long-Term Investment:

- **Perennial Yield:** Blueberry bushes can produce fruit for many years with proper care, offering a long-term return on the initial investment of time and resources.

8. Emotional Well-being:

- **Stress Relief:** Gardening, including tending to blueberry plants, is known to reduce stress and promote mental well-being through the therapeutic aspects of nurturing plants and being in nature.

The benefits of growing blueberries are far-reaching, touching upon health, financial, environmental, social, and personal aspects. Whether cultivated on a small scale in backyard gardens or as part of larger agricultural enterprises, the act of nurturing these bushes and harvesting their delicious fruits offers a myriad of rewards beyond the mere satisfaction of a bountiful harvest.

CHAPTER 2

Types of Blueberries

2.1 Highbush Blueberries

Highbush blueberries (Vaccinium corymbosum) are one of the most widely cultivated types of blueberries, favored for their size, flavor, and adaptability to various growing conditions. Here's a detailed overview:

Characteristics:

- **Size and Growth:** Highbush blueberry bushes are relatively large, reaching heights between 4 to 8 feet tall. They can spread to about 3 to 6 feet wide, creating substantial bushes with a dense growth habit.

- **Foliage:** The foliage is typically a vibrant green during the growing season, turning to shades of red or yellow in autumn, adding ornamental value to gardens.

- **Berries:** The berries are relatively large, round, and often have a sweet, mildly tart flavor. They come in various shades of blue and can range from mild to very flavorful, depending on the cultivar.

Cultivars and Varieties:

- **Northern Highbush:** Well-suited for colder climates, these varieties include 'Bluecrop,' 'Jersey,' and 'Patriot,' among others. They typically have a chilling requirement and thrive in regions with cold winters.

- **Southern Highbush:** Bred to tolerate milder winters, these varieties, such as 'O'Neal' and 'Sunshine Blue,' are adapted to warmer climates and have a lower chilling requirement.

Growing Conditions:

- **Climate:** Highbush blueberries thrive in temperate climates. While they prefer cooler regions, certain cultivars are bred to withstand warmer climates as well.

- **Soil and pH:** They prefer acidic soil with a pH range between 4.5 to 5.5. Well-draining, loamy soil with organic matter is optimal for their growth.

Care and Maintenance:

- **Pruning:** Regular pruning is essential for highbush blueberries to encourage new growth, remove dead wood, and maintain shape.

- **Fertilization:** Applying acidic fertilizers rich in nutrients like ammonium sulfate helps maintain optimal soil conditions.

- **Watering:** Consistent moisture is crucial, especially during the fruiting season, to ensure proper berry development.

Uses:

- **Culinary Delights:** Highbush blueberries are ideal for fresh eating, baking, making jams, preserves, and incorporating into various culinary creations due to their larger size and flavorful taste.

- **Landscape Ornament:** Beyond their fruit-bearing potential, highbush blueberry bushes can be used as ornamental shrubs in landscaping, offering aesthetic appeal with their foliage and seasonal color changes.

Highbush blueberries are prized for their delicious fruits and adaptability to different climates, making them a popular choice among home gardeners and commercial growers alike. Understanding their specific needs and growth patterns is key to successfully cultivating these flavorful berries.

2.2 Lowbush Blueberries

Lowbush blueberries (Vaccinium angustifolium) are a distinct variety known for their smaller stature, hardiness, and suitability for various landscapes. Here's a detailed overview:

Characteristics:

- **Size and Growth:** Lowbush blueberries are compact, typically reaching heights of 6 to 24 inches, forming dense, spreading mats due to their rhizomatous growth habit.

- **Foliage:** The foliage is characterized by small, narrow leaves that turn vibrant shades of red, orange, and yellow during the fall, adding ornamental value.

- **Berries:** These blueberries are smaller in size compared to highbush varieties, but they pack a powerful, sweet-tart flavor. They're often used for processing into jams, jellies, and other products.

Cultivars and Varieties:

- **Wild Varieties:** Lowbush blueberries are often found in the wild across North America, particularly in regions with acidic, sandy soil, such as parts of New England and Canada.

- **Cultivated Varieties:** Some cultivated varieties, like 'Top Hat' and 'Patriot,' are bred for compact growth, making them suitable for container gardening or smaller spaces.

Growing Conditions:

- **Climate:** Lowbush blueberries are exceptionally cold-hardy and thrive in northern climates, enduring harsh winters.

- **Soil and pH:** They prefer acidic, well-draining, sandy soil with a pH ranging between 4.0 to 5.0. Sandy or rocky soils are often conducive to their growth.

Care and Maintenance:

- **Pruning:** Pruning lowbush blueberries involves removing dead or damaged wood and thinning out older canes to encourage new growth.

- **Wildlife Management:** Protection from birds and other wildlife may be necessary, as these berries are popular among various animals.

Uses:

- **Culinary Applications:** While smaller in size, lowbush blueberries are prized for their intense flavor, making them ideal for jams, preserves, and baking, imparting a robust taste to dishes.

- **Landscaping:** Due to their low growth habit and beautiful fall foliage, lowbush blueberries are often used in landscaping, particularly in naturalized settings, borders, or rock gardens.

Commercial Harvesting:

- **Wild Harvesting:** In regions where they grow abundantly, lowbush blueberries are commercially harvested by hand or with small rakes, contributing to the production of blueberry-based products.

Lowbush blueberries, known for their hardiness, delectable flavor, and ornamental qualities, are a valuable addition to both natural landscapes and cultivated gardens. Understanding their preference for acidic soil and their unique growth habits is key to successfully growing these flavorful berries.

2.3 Rabbiteye Blueberries

Rabbiteye blueberries (Vaccinium ashei) are a variety highly regarded for their adaptability to warmer climates and their resilience against certain pests and diseases. Here's a comprehensive overview of these blueberries:

Characteristics:

- **Size and Growth:** Rabbiteye blueberry bushes are relatively large, typically reaching heights of 6 to 10 feet, with some varieties growing even taller. They have an upright growth habit.

- **Foliage:** The foliage is typically a glossy green during the growing season, turning shades of red and purple in the fall, enhancing their ornamental appeal.

- **Berries:** Rabbiteye blueberries are known for their medium to large-sized berries that are often firm, sweet, and slightly tart, making them excellent for fresh eating and processing.

Cultivars and Varieties:

- **Cultivated Varieties:** Varieties such as 'Climax,' 'Premier,' and 'Tifblue' are among the popular rabbiteye blueberry cultivars, each with unique characteristics, including flavor profile and harvest time.

Growing Conditions:

- **Climate:** Rabbiteye blueberries thrive in warm climates, particularly in regions with hot summers and mild winters, such as the southeastern United States.

- **Soil and pH:** They prefer well-draining, acidic soil with a pH ranging between 4.0 to 5.5. Sandy or loamy soils are often suitable for their growth.

Care and Maintenance:

- **Pruning:** Pruning rabbiteye blueberries involves removing dead or weak wood, shaping the bush, and thinning out crowded branches to increase airflow and sun exposure.

- **Irrigation:** Adequate watering, especially during dry periods and fruit development, is crucial for optimal berry production.

Uses:

- **Fresh Consumption:** Rabbiteye blueberries are delicious when eaten fresh, boasting a balance of sweetness and slight acidity.

- **Processing:** Their firm texture makes them well-suited for various processing methods, including freezing, canning, and use in baked goods.

Commercial Cultivation:

- **Commercial Farms:** Rabbiteye blueberries are cultivated on a larger scale in commercial farms in regions where they thrive, contributing significantly to the blueberry market.

- **U-Pick Farms:** Many farms allow visitors to pick their own rabbiteye blueberries during the harvest season, offering an engaging agritourism experience.

Rabbiteye blueberries, prized for their adaptability to warmer climates and their flavorful, versatile berries, play a significant role in both commercial agriculture and home gardening. Understanding their specific needs and growth patterns is essential for successfully cultivating these robust and delicious berries.

CHAPTER 3

Climate and Soil Requirements

3.1 Ideal Climate for Blueberries

Blueberries have specific climate preferences crucial for their growth and fruit production. The ideal climate varies slightly depending on the type of blueberry but generally includes these considerations:

Highbush Blueberries:

- **Temperature:** Highbush blueberries thrive in regions with cool to moderate temperatures. They typically prefer regions with winter chilling hours between 1,000 to 1,200 hours below 45°F (7°C).

- **Hardiness Zones:** They grow well in USDA hardiness zones 4 to 7, but specific cultivars can extend this range slightly, with some tolerant to zones 3 and 8.

Lowbush Blueberries:

- **Temperature:** Lowbush blueberries are exceptionally cold-hardy and flourish in colder climates with cooler summers. They can endure harsh winter conditions and are often found in regions with low winter temperatures.

- **Hardiness Zones:** They are commonly found in USDA hardiness zones 3 to 6.

Rabbiteye Blueberries:

- **Temperature:** Rabbiteye blueberries thrive in warmer climates, particularly regions with hot summers and mild winters. They are well-suited for areas with high summer temperatures.

- **Hardiness Zones:** They grow best in USDA hardiness zones 7 to 9, although some cultivars might extend into zone 6 with proper care.

Blueberries require a specific number of chilling hours during winter to break dormancy and set fruit properly. However, some cultivars within each type have been bred to adapt to a broader range of climates. Understanding the particular climatic needs of the specific blueberry variety you intend to grow is essential for successful cultivation.

3.2 Soil Preparation and pH Levels

Preparing the soil and maintaining the appropriate pH levels are critical factors for successful blueberry cultivation. Here's a detailed overview:

Soil Preparation:

1. **Texture and Drainage:** Blueberries thrive in well-draining soils. Sandy or loamy soils are often preferred over heavy clay soils to prevent waterlogging, which can harm blueberry roots.

2. **Organic Matter:** Incorporating organic matter, such as peat moss, compost, or pine bark, into the soil improves its structure and aids in moisture retention without sacrificing drainage.

3. **Weed Control:** Clearing the planting area of weeds and grasses is crucial before planting

blueberries. Mulching helps control weeds and maintains soil moisture.

pH Levels:

1. **Acidic Soil:** Blueberries have a specific need for acidic soil. They thrive in soil with a pH level ranging between 4.0 to 5.5. The ideal pH may vary slightly depending on the blueberry variety.

2. **Soil Testing:** Conduct soil tests before planting to determine the soil's pH and nutrient levels. This helps in adjusting the soil to meet blueberries' pH requirements.

3. **Acidifying Agents:** To lower pH levels, sulfur or acidic fertilizers can be added to the soil based on the soil test recommendations. These amendments should be applied well in advance of planting to allow time for the soil pH to adjust.

Planting Considerations:

1. **Raised Beds:** Creating raised beds or mounds can help ensure proper drainage, especially in areas with less than ideal soil conditions.

2. **Spacing:** Blueberry plants should be spaced adequately to allow for proper airflow and sunlight penetration, generally around 4 to 6 feet apart in rows with 8 to 10 feet between rows.

3. **Planting Depth:** When planting blueberries, ensure they are set at the same depth as they were in their nursery containers. Planting too deeply can hinder growth.

Maintenance:

1. **Mulching:** Applying mulch, such as pine needles, wood chips, or sawdust, helps maintain soil moisture, suppress weeds, and gradually acidifies the soil as it decomposes.

2. **Fertilization:** Blueberries have specific nutrient requirements. Fertilizers designed for acid-loving plants, like ammonium sulfate or specialized blueberry fertilizers, can be applied according to the plant's needs and soil test results.

Ensuring proper soil preparation, maintaining the correct pH levels, and providing adequate care are vital for blueberries to establish healthy root systems and thrive, leading to robust growth and a bountiful harvest.

CHAPTER 4

Choosing the Right Varieties

4.1 Considerations for Variety Selection

When selecting blueberry varieties for cultivation, several key considerations can guide your choice:

Climate Suitability:

- **Chilling Hours:** Consider the chilling hours required by the variety. Some need more cold hours in winter to break dormancy and produce fruit, while others are suited for milder climates.

Size and Growth Habit:

- **Bush Size:** Assess the space available and the desired bush size. Highbush blueberries tend to grow taller, while lowbush and rabbiteye varieties have different growth habits, staying more compact.

Harvest Time and Yield:

- **Ripening Period:** Opt for varieties that span different ripening periods to enjoy a longer harvest season.

- **Yield:** Some varieties produce larger yields than others. Consider your consumption needs and whether you plan to preserve or share the harvest.

Flavor and Use:

- **Taste Profile:** Different varieties offer varying flavor profiles, from sweeter to more tart. Consider personal preferences and intended culinary uses.

- **Fresh vs. Processing:** Certain types are better suited for fresh consumption, while others hold up well for processing into jams, preserves, or baking.

Pest and Disease Resistance:

- **Resistance Traits:** Some cultivars exhibit resistance or tolerance to certain pests or diseases prevalent in your region. Select varieties known for their resistance to common issues in your area.

Soil and Climate Adaptability:

- **pH Tolerance:** Certain varieties might be more adaptable to specific soil pH ranges.

- **Climate Adaptability:** Consider if the variety is well-suited to your region's climate, whether it's colder or warmer.

Local Recommendations and Experience:

- **Consult Experts:** Seek advice from local nurseries, agricultural extension offices, or experienced growers in your area. They can provide valuable insights into successful varieties for your specific locale.

Popular Varieties and Reviews:

- **Research and Reviews:** Look into reviews, gardening forums, and publications to learn about popular and well-regarded varieties among gardeners and growers in your region.

Ultimately, the ideal blueberry variety depends on your specific growing conditions, preferences, and intended use of the berries. Assessing these considerations will help you select varieties that align best with your goals and ensure a successful blueberry harvest.

4.2 Recommended Blueberry Varieties

Highbush Blueberries:

1. **'Bluecrop':** Known for its high yield, large berries, and excellent flavor, 'Bluecrop' is a popular choice for both home gardens and commercial cultivation.

2. **'Patriot':** This variety is prized for its cold-hardiness, making it suitable for northern climates. It produces flavorful berries and has good disease resistance.

3. **'Legacy':** 'Legacy' is recognized for its sweet-tart flavor, good yields, and tolerance to various soil types, making it adaptable to different conditions.

Lowbush Blueberries:

1. **'Top Hat':** A compact variety ideal for smaller spaces or container gardening, 'Top Hat' produces

small but flavorful berries and is well-suited for colder climates.

2. **'Patriot':** While 'Patriot' is primarily a highbush variety, it's also known for its compact growth, making it suitable for those seeking a smaller blueberry bush.

Rabbiteye Blueberries:

1. **'Climax':** Renowned for its sweet and flavorful berries, 'Climax' is an early-season rabbiteye variety that performs well in warmer climates.

2. **'Tifblue':** A mid to late-season variety, 'Tifblue' is favored for its large, firm berries and adaptability to various soil conditions.

These recommended varieties offer a range of flavors, adaptability to different climates, and specific growth characteristics suited for various gardening preferences. However, it's crucial to verify the suitability of these varieties based on your specific climate, soil conditions, and local recommendations before making your selection. Consulting local experts or nurseries can provide tailored advice for the best blueberry varieties in your region.

CHAPTER 5

Planting Blueberries

5.1 Best Time to Plant

The best time to plant blueberries depends on various factors including your climate, the type of blueberry, and the nursery stock available. However, there are general guidelines for optimal planting times:

Highbush Blueberries:

- **Fall or Early Spring:** In moderate climates, planting in fall (September to November) allows roots to establish before winter. In colder regions, early spring (March to April) after the last frost is suitable.

Lowbush Blueberries:

- **Early Spring:** Lowbush varieties are best planted in early spring (March to April) to allow them to establish before the growing season begins.

Rabbiteye Blueberries:

- **Late Fall to Early Spring:** Rabbiteye blueberries can be planted in late fall (November) in warmer climates or in early spring (March to April) when the soil is workable.

Considerations for Planting:

1. **Soil Conditions:** Ensure the soil is well-prepared with the appropriate pH levels before planting.

2. **Weather Conditions:** Avoid planting during extreme weather conditions, such as excessively hot or dry periods, as young plants may struggle to establish in such conditions.

3. **Plant Health:** Choose healthy, nursery-grown plants with well-developed root systems for optimal growth.

4. **Spacing:** Plant blueberries according to recommended spacing for the specific type and variety. Typically, they should be spaced about 4 to 6 feet apart in rows.

5. **Planting Depth:** Set plants at the same depth they were in the nursery container, making sure the root ball is adequately covered with soil.

6. **Mulching and Watering:** Mulch around the plants to retain moisture and suppress weeds. Water thoroughly after planting to help the roots settle and reduce transplant shock.

Always check your local climate and the specific needs of the blueberry variety you're planting to determine the most suitable time. Adequate preparation and proper planting techniques significantly contribute to the successful establishment and growth of blueberry plants.

5.2 Spacing and Layout

The spacing and layout of blueberry plants play a crucial role in their growth, productivity, and ease of maintenance. Here's a guide on spacing and layout considerations:

Spacing:

1. **Highbush Blueberries:**

   - **Between Plants:** Generally, highbush blueberries should be spaced about 4 to 6 feet apart in rows.

   - **Between Rows:** Rows of highbush blueberries should have a spacing of 8 to 10 feet between them, allowing adequate space for maintenance and harvesting.

2. **Lowbush Blueberries:**

   - **Spacing for Mats:** Lowbush blueberries tend to form spreading mats. Allow about 2 to 3 feet between plants within the mat and space mats approximately 3 to 4 feet apart.

3. **Rabbiteye Blueberries:**

   - **Between Plants:** Rabbiteye blueberries benefit from a spacing of about 6 to 10 feet apart in rows.

   - **Between Rows:** Maintain a distance of 10 to 12 feet between rows to accommodate their larger growth.

Layout Considerations:

1. **Orientation:** Plant rows of blueberries in a north-south direction to ensure even sunlight exposure throughout the day.

2. **Access Paths:** Designate pathways between rows for easy access during maintenance, harvesting, and pest management.

3. **Grouping Varieties:** If planting multiple blueberry varieties, consider grouping similar varieties together to facilitate care and harvesting. This can also aid in cross-pollination, especially for certain types that require it.

4. **Aesthetic Considerations:** Blueberries can be integrated into ornamental landscapes. Consider their visual appeal, especially during different seasons with their foliage and fruit color variations.

Proper spacing and layout are vital for ensuring adequate airflow, sunlight exposure, and ease of management. They also allow the plants to reach their full potential, resulting in healthier growth and higher yields of delicious blueberries. Adjustments to spacing might be necessary based on specific variety requirements and available space in your garden or orchard.

5.3 Planting Process Step-by-Step

1. Choose the Right Location:

- Select a site with well-draining soil and adequate sunlight (at least 6-8 hours of direct sunlight daily).

- Ensure the soil pH is within the ideal range of 4.0 to 5.5 for blueberries.

2. Prepare the Soil:

- Test the soil to determine its pH and nutrient levels.

- Incorporate organic matter like peat moss or compost to improve soil structure and acidity if needed.

- Clear the planting area of weeds and grasses.

3. Obtain Healthy Plants:

- Purchase healthy, disease-free blueberry plants from a reputable nursery.

- Consider the variety suited to your climate and soil conditions.

4. Planting:

- **Digging Holes:** Dig holes that are twice the width of the root ball and just as deep.

- **Spacing:** Space the plants according to the recommended distance for the specific type of blueberry.

- **Planting Depth:** Place the blueberry plant in the hole, ensuring the top of the root ball is level with the ground surface.

- **Backfilling:** Gently fill the hole with soil, firming it around the roots but avoid compacting excessively.

- **Mulching:** Apply a layer of mulch around the plant, leaving space around the stem to prevent moisture accumulation.

5. Watering:

- Water the newly planted blueberries thoroughly to settle the soil around the roots.

- Ensure consistent moisture, especially during the establishment phase.

6. Care After Planting:

- **Fertilization:** Apply a balanced fertilizer according to the specific needs of the blueberries and soil test recommendations.

- **Pruning:** Initially, prune any damaged or dead branches. More extensive pruning can be done in subsequent years.

7. Maintenance:

- Regularly check soil moisture and water as needed, especially during dry spells.

- Monitor for pests, diseases, and weeds, and take appropriate measures for management.

- Provide protection from birds if necessary, during fruiting season.

8. Patience and Observation:

- Blueberries take time to establish and produce substantial yields. Be patient and observe their growth regularly.

Following these steps and providing proper care and maintenance after planting will help your blueberry plants establish healthy root systems and lead to successful

growth and fruit production in the seasons
to come.

CHAPTER 6

Care and Maintenance

6.1 Watering Guidelines

Proper watering is crucial for the health and productivity of blueberry plants. Here are some watering guidelines to ensure optimal growth:

1. Consistent Moisture:

- Blueberries require consistently moist soil, especially during their active growth periods, flowering, and fruit development.

- Aim to keep the soil evenly moist but not waterlogged. Soggy soil can lead to root rot, while dry soil can stress the plants.

2. Frequency:

- Water deeply and thoroughly, ensuring the entire root zone gets moisture.

- In general, blueberries need about 1 to 2 inches of water per week, including rainfall. Adjust based on weather conditions and soil moisture levels.

3. Timing:

- Water in the morning to allow foliage to dry during the day, reducing the risk of fungal diseases.

- Avoid watering late in the day or at night to prevent prolonged moisture on the leaves.

4. Drip Irrigation or Soaker Hoses:

- Drip irrigation or soaker hoses are excellent watering methods for blueberries as they deliver water directly to the root zone, minimizing moisture on the leaves.

5. Mulching:

- Apply a layer of mulch around the plants to retain moisture, regulate soil temperature, and reduce water evaporation. Mulch also helps suppress weeds that could compete for moisture.

6. Soil Monitoring:

- Regularly check soil moisture levels by probing the soil around the root zone. Water when the top inch of soil feels dry.

7. Consideration for Containers:

- If growing blueberries in containers, monitor soil moisture more frequently as containers tend to dry out faster than garden soil.

8. Adjusting for Seasonal Changes:

- Increase watering during hot, dry periods or when the plants are flowering and fruiting.

- Reduce watering in cooler weather or during dormancy in late fall and winter, but ensure the plants don't completely dry out.

Consistent and appropriate watering practices play a vital role in blueberry plant health. It's essential to strike a balance, avoiding both overwatering and underwatering, to ensure robust growth, flowering, and fruit production.

6.2 Fertilizing Blueberries

1. **Acidic Fertilizer:** Blueberries thrive in acidic soil. Choose a fertilizer specifically formulated for acid-loving plants or those designed for blueberries.

2. **Timing:** Apply fertilizer in early spring before new growth begins, typically around March or April. Avoid late-season fertilization, as it can stimulate late growth vulnerable to frost damage.

3. **Quantity:** Follow package instructions for the recommended dosage based on the age and size of the blueberry bushes. Over-fertilizing can harm the plants.

4. **Spread Out Application:** Divide the total recommended amount into multiple applications throughout the growing season to provide a steady supply of nutrients.

5. **Organic Options:** Organic fertilizers such as compost, pine bark, or well-rotted manure can be used to improve soil structure and provide slow-release nutrients.

6. **Soil pH Monitoring:** Periodically check the soil pH to ensure it remains within the ideal range of 4.0 to 5.5 for optimal nutrient uptake.

6.3 Pruning Techniques

1. **Annual Pruning:** Regular pruning is essential for blueberries to maintain plant health, shape the bushes, and encourage fruit production.

2. **Timing:** Prune during late winter or early spring before new growth begins. Remove dead, damaged, or diseased branches and thin out crowded growth.

3. **Thinning:** Remove some of the older, less productive canes to allow sunlight and air circulation, promoting the growth of new canes and better fruiting.

4. **Pruning Style for Types:**

   - **Highbush:** Prune to maintain a vase-like shape, removing low growth and inward-growing branches.

- **Rabbiteye:** Prune to shape the bush and remove dead wood and crowded branches.

5. **Minimal Cutting:** Avoid excessive pruning, as blueberries produce fruit on older wood. Aim to remove about 20% of the older wood each year.

6. **Pruning Tools:** Use sharp, clean pruning shears or loppers to make clean cuts without causing unnecessary damage to the plants.

Regular fertilizing and proper pruning play a crucial role in blueberry plant health, ensuring they receive the necessary nutrients and maintenance for optimal growth, fruit production, and overall longevity. Adjust fertilization and pruning techniques based on specific variety requirements and plant health indicators.

6.4 Mulching Tips

Mulching is a beneficial practice for blueberries, providing several advantages in maintaining soil moisture, suppressing weeds, regulating soil temperature, and contributing to soil acidity. Here are some mulching tips specifically tailored for blueberries:

1. Ideal Mulch Types:

- **Organic Materials:** Use organic mulches such as pine bark, pine needles (also known as pine straw), wood chips, sawdust, or compost. These materials gradually decompose, enriching the soil with organic matter.

2. Application Guidelines:

- **Depth:** Apply a layer of mulch around 2 to 4 inches thick around the base of blueberry plants. Ensure the mulch doesn't touch the main stem to prevent excess moisture accumulation or potential rot.

3. Benefits of Mulching:

- **Moisture Retention:** Mulch helps retain soil moisture, crucial for blueberries that require consistently moist but well-draining soil.

- **Weed Suppression:** A thick layer of mulch helps suppress weeds, reducing competition for nutrients and moisture.

- **Soil Temperature Regulation:** Mulch acts as insulation, moderating soil temperatures and protecting the roots during extreme weather conditions.

- **Acidification:** Certain organic mulches, like pine needles or pine bark, can gradually acidify the soil, which is beneficial for blueberries that thrive in acidic conditions.

4. Replenishment and Maintenance:

- **Regular Checks:** Monitor the mulch layer regularly. Over time,

organic mulches break down and
may need replenishing.

- **Annual Top-Ups:** Add a fresh
layer of mulch annually or as
needed, especially after
decomposition or in areas where
the layer has thinned out.

5. Mulch Spread:

- **Extended Coverage:** Extend the
mulch layer beyond the immediate
root zone of the blueberry bushes to
prevent weed growth and maintain
consistent soil moisture in a wider
area.

6. Considerations:

- **Pine Needle Mulch:** Pine needles
are particularly beneficial for
blueberries due to their acidic
nature, contributing to the preferred
soil pH levels.

- **Avoid Compactness:** While
applying mulch, ensure it remains

loose and airy around the base of
the plants to allow proper airflow to
the root zone.

Applying and maintaining an appropriate
layer of mulch around blueberries aids in
their overall health and contributes to an
environment conducive to their growth
and productivity. Adjust mulching
practices based on the specific needs of the
blueberry variety and local climate
conditions.

CHAPTER 7

Pest and Disease Management

7.1 Common Pests Affecting Blueberries

Several pests can affect blueberry plants, potentially impacting their health and fruit production. Here are some common pests to watch out for:

1. Spotted Wing Drosophila (SWD):

- This fruit fly lays eggs in ripening berries, causing them to spoil. Larvae feed inside the fruit, making it susceptible to rot.

2. Blueberry Maggot:

- The larvae of this fly burrow into blueberries, causing them to become soft and unmarketable.

Infested berries might have visible
entry holes.

3. Blueberry Gall Midge:

- Larvae of this midge feed on
  developing flower buds, causing
  them to swell and distort, impacting
  fruit production.

4. Japanese Beetle:

- Both adults and larvae can cause
  damage. Adults feed on leaves,
  causing skeletonized foliage, while
  larvae feed on roots, affecting plant
  health.

5. Aphids:

- Aphids suck sap from leaves and
  stems, causing curling or distortion
  of foliage. They can also spread
  viruses.

6. Thrips:

- Thrips feed on flower buds and
  leaves, leaving scars or causing

deformation, leading to reduced
fruit quality.

7. Spider Mites:

- These tiny pests feed on plant juices, causing yellow stippling or discoloration on leaves, which can affect photosynthesis.

8. Blueberry Stem Gall Wasp:

- This pest causes galls or swellings on stems, impacting plant vigor and growth.

9. Scale Insects:

- Scales feed on plant sap, causing yellowing of leaves, weakened growth, and in severe cases, plant decline.

10. Cranberry Fruitworm:

- The larvae feed on flower buds and developing berries, leading to fruit damage.

Monitoring and Management:

- Regularly inspect plants for signs of pest infestation, especially during vulnerable growth stages.

- Use insecticidal soaps, neem oil, or botanical insecticides as natural control methods.

- Employ cultural practices like pruning, proper plant spacing, and removing and destroying infested plant parts to reduce pest populations.

- Biological control methods using predatory insects or nematodes can also help manage certain pests.

Early detection and a combination of preventative measures and targeted interventions are essential for effectively managing pest issues in blueberries while minimizing the use of chemical pesticides.

7.2 Diseases and Their Prevention

Blueberries are susceptible to various diseases that can impact plant health and reduce fruit yield. Here are some common diseases affecting blueberries and preventive measures:

1. Mummy Berry (Monilinia vaccinii-corymbosi):

- Symptoms include shriveled, discolored berries. Infected berries drop prematurely, and the fungus produces resting spores (mummies) on the ground.

- Prevention:

    - Apply fungicides preventatively during bloom to protect against infection.

    - Remove and destroy infected mummified berries promptly to reduce spore production.

2. Powdery Mildew (Microsphaera penicillata):

- Appears as a white powdery growth on leaves and shoots, causing leaf distortion and reduced fruit quality.

- Prevention:

    - Maintain good air circulation by proper plant spacing and pruning to reduce humidity around the plants.

    - Apply fungicides preventatively during the growing season.

3. Phytophthora Root Rot (Phytophthora cinnamomi):

- Causes root decay, leading to stunted growth, wilting, and eventual plant death.

- Prevention:

- Ensure proper soil drainage and avoid waterlogged conditions.

- Plant blueberries in raised beds or mounds to improve drainage.

- Use resistant varieties if available.

4. Anthracnose (Colletotrichum gloeosporioides):

- Symptoms include small, sunken lesions on fruit, twig dieback, and leaf spots.

- Prevention:

  - Prune out infected twigs and branches during dormancy to reduce disease spread.

  - Apply fungicides as a preventive measure during the growing season.

5. Botrytis Blight (Botrytis cinerea):

- Leads to fruit rot, especially in wet conditions during flowering and fruiting.

- Prevention:

  - Promote good air circulation by proper plant spacing and pruning.

  - Remove and destroy infected plant material promptly.

  - Apply fungicides during bloom and fruit development if necessary.

6. Bacterial Blight (Pseudomonas syringae):

- Symptoms include water-soaked lesions on leaves and stems, leading to dieback.

- Prevention:

  - Avoid overhead irrigation to reduce moisture on foliage.

- Prune out infected branches and practice good sanitation.

7. Virus Diseases (Various):

- Virus infections can cause various symptoms like leaf mottling, stunting, and reduced fruit quality.

- Prevention:

    - Use virus-free planting material.

    - Control aphid vectors that spread viruses by monitoring and managing aphid populations.

Good cultural practices, such as proper sanitation, maintaining plant health, using disease-resistant varieties, and timely application of fungicides or other control measures, are crucial for preventing and managing diseases in blueberries. Regular monitoring and early intervention can significantly reduce disease impact.

CHAPTER 8

Harvesting Blueberries

8.1 Signs of Ripeness

Determining the optimal time to harvest blueberries involves observing several key indicators that signify ripeness. Here are signs to look for:

1. Color:

- Blueberries typically change color as they ripen, transitioning from green to shades of blue or purple, depending on the variety. Ripe berries often have a deep, uniform color without any green or red tones.

2. Size and Plumpness:

- Ripe blueberries are plump, round, and generally larger than unripe ones. They should feel full and firm to the touch without being too soft or squishy.

3. Texture:

- Gently touch the berries to check for firmness. Ripe blueberries have a firm texture but yield slightly to pressure.

4. Taste and Flavor:

- The most reliable indicator is taste. Ripe blueberries have a sweet, juicy flavor with the characteristic blueberry taste. Taste-testing a few berries can confirm their ripeness.

5. Cluster Ripening:

- Blueberries in a cluster don't all ripen simultaneously. Check individual berries within a cluster for ripeness and pick those that are

fully mature while leaving the
unripe ones to continue ripening.

6. Harvest Period:

- Blueberries ripen over several
  weeks, so monitor the plants
  regularly during the harvest season.
  Pick berries as they become ripe to
  prevent overripening or spoilage.

7. Appearance of Fruit Cluster:

- An entire cluster won't ripen
  uniformly. Look for clusters where
  most berries have reached the
  desired color and size for
  harvesting.

8. Ease of Removal:

- Ripe blueberries should come off
  easily when gently tugged. If they
  resist or are difficult to detach from
  the stem, they might not be fully
  ripe.

Observing these signs collectively helps
determine the ideal time for harvesting

blueberries. Aim for berries that display a
rich color, plumpness, and a sweet taste
for the best flavor and quality.

8.2 Harvesting Techniques

Harvesting blueberries requires care to
ensure the best quality and to preserve the
plants for future growth. Here are some
techniques to harvest blueberries:

1. Gentle Handling:

- Blueberries are delicate. Handle
  them with care to avoid bruising or
  damaging the fruit and the plant.

2. Handpicking:

- Using your fingers, gently pluck
  ripe blueberries from the stem.
  Hold the cluster with one hand and
  use the other to pick individual ripe
  berries. Ripe berries should easily
  separate from the stem with a
  gentle tug.

3. Use a Rake or Comb:

- For larger-scale harvests, consider using a specialized blueberry rake or comb. Gently rake the berries off the bushes, allowing them to fall onto a catching surface like a tarp or a tray.

4. Repeat Harvesting:

- Blueberries ripen over time, so plan for multiple harvesting sessions. Check the plants regularly, typically every few days, during the harvest season to collect ripe berries while leaving the unripe ones to mature.

5. Timing of Harvest:

- Harvest blueberries during the cooler parts of the day, such as early morning or late afternoon, to prevent the berries from becoming too warm or soft while picking.

6. Proper Storage:

- After harvesting, store blueberries in a cool place or refrigerate them promptly to maintain freshness. Avoid stacking or overcrowding the berries to prevent crushing or bruising.

7. Harvesting Containers:

- Use shallow containers to collect harvested blueberries. Avoid filling the containers too high to prevent crushing the bottom layers of berries.

8. Sanitation:

- Ensure cleanliness during harvesting. Wash hands before picking and use clean containers to avoid contamination.

9. Field Etiquette:

- When harvesting from U-pick farms or community gardens, follow guidelines provided by the farm or garden regarding picking techniques, payment, and etiquette.

Following these techniques not only ensures a successful harvest but also helps maintain the quality of the blueberries and the health of the plants for continued growth and future yields.

8.3 Post-Harvest Care

Post-harvest care is crucial for maintaining the quality and extending the shelf life of freshly harvested blueberries. Here are steps for effective post-harvest care:

1. Cool Quickly:

- Blueberries should be cooled as soon as possible after harvesting to preserve their freshness. Transfer them to a cool environment or refrigerate promptly.

2. Handling and Sorting:

- Gently handle the blueberries to avoid damaging the fruit. Remove any damaged, overripe, or moldy berries.

3. Cleaning:

- Rinse blueberries gently under cold running water just before use. Pat them dry with paper towels or allow them to air dry.

4. Storage Conditions:

- Store blueberries in perforated plastic bags or containers in the refrigerator. Properly stored blueberries can remain fresh for about a week.

5. Avoid Compression:

- Store blueberries in a single layer or loosely packed to prevent crushing or bruising, which can lead to spoilage.

6. Freezing for Long-Term Storage:

- If not using blueberries immediately, consider freezing them for longer-term storage. Spread them in a single layer on a baking sheet and freeze before transferring to airtight containers or bags.

7. Proper Humidity:

- Maintain a higher humidity level in the refrigerator (around 90%) for stored blueberries to prevent dehydration.

8. Check and Remove Spoiled Berries:

- Periodically check stored blueberries for any signs of spoilage. Remove any spoiled berries promptly to prevent the spread of mold to others.

9. Use in Various Culinary Preparations:

- Enjoy blueberries fresh or use them in various recipes such as

smoothies, jams, pies, or baked
goods.

By following these post-harvest care steps,
you can prolong the shelf life and maintain
the quality of freshly harvested
blueberries, ensuring you get the most out
of your harvest both in flavor and
nutritional value.

CHAPTER 9

Troubleshooting Common Issues

9.1 Yellowing Leaves

Yellowing leaves in blueberry plants can be indicative of various issues, including nutritional deficiencies, pest infestations, diseases, or environmental stress. Here are potential causes and solutions for yellowing leaves in blueberries:

1. Nutritional Deficiencies:

- **Iron Deficiency (Chlorosis):** This is a common issue in blueberries due to their preference for acidic soil.

  - Solution: Adjust the soil pH to the recommended range of 4.0 to 5.5 using amendments like sulfur or iron sulfate. Apply chelated iron or iron-rich fertilizers if needed.

2. Watering Problems:

- **Overwatering or Waterlogged Soil:** Excessive moisture can lead to root suffocation and nutrient uptake issues.

  - Solution: Improve drainage by amending soil or raising beds. Adjust watering practices to ensure the soil is consistently moist but not waterlogged.

3. Pest Infestations:

- **Root Weevil Larvae or Other Pests:** Larvae feeding on roots can cause yellowing leaves and overall decline.

  - Solution: Inspect the root zone for pests. Use appropriate insecticides or beneficial nematodes for control if infestations are confirmed.

4. Diseases:

- **Root Rot or Phytophthora:** These diseases can cause yellowing leaves due to root damage.

  - Solution: Improve soil drainage, avoid overwatering, and use disease-resistant varieties. Remove affected plants and avoid planting new ones in the same area.

5. Environmental Stress:

- **Heat Stress or Sunburn:** High temperatures or intense sunlight can stress plants, leading to leaf discoloration.

  - Solution: Provide shade during the hottest parts of the day, especially for young or sensitive plants. Mulch around the base of plants to regulate soil temperature.

6. Winter Damage:

- **Winter Burn or Cold Injury:** Cold winter temperatures can cause leaf damage and yellowing.

    - Solution: Protect plants from extreme cold with covers or mulch, and prune damaged branches in early spring.

7. pH Imbalance:

- **Alkaline Soil:** Blueberries prefer acidic soil, and high pH levels can lead to nutrient uptake issues.

    - Solution: Adjust soil pH by adding acidifying agents or amendments to achieve the optimal pH range.

8. Overfertilization:

- **Excessive Nitrogen:** Too much nitrogen can lead to leaf discoloration and affect overall plant health.

  - Solution: Avoid excessive fertilization, especially with nitrogen-rich fertilizers.

Identifying the specific cause of yellowing leaves in blueberries involves careful observation and assessment of environmental conditions, soil health, and possible pest or disease presence. Tailor solutions based on the underlying issue to restore the plant's health and vigor. Consulting local gardening experts or extension services can provide targeted advice for specific issues in your area.

9.2 Poor Fruit Production

Environmental Factors:

1. **Climate and Weather Conditions:**

- Inadequate sunlight, extreme temperatures, or unseasonal weather patterns can negatively impact fruit production. Plants may require specific temperature ranges and photoperiods for optimal growth and flowering.

2. **Soil Quality and Composition:**

   - Poor soil fertility, improper pH levels, or insufficient organic matter can hinder nutrient absorption by plants. This, in turn, affects their ability to set fruit and undergo successful pollination.

3. **Watering Practices:**

   - Irregular watering, overwatering, or underwatering can lead to stress in plants, affecting their reproductive processes. Consistent and appropriate irrigation is crucial for maintaining optimal soil moisture.

4. **Pollination Issues:**

   - Lack of pollinators, such as bees, or poor pollination efficiency can result in low fruit set. Some plants require cross-pollination, and factors affecting pollinator populations can have a direct impact on fruit production.

5. **Disease and Pest Infestations:**

   - Pathogens and pests can attack the plant's reproductive organs, leading to flower drop, reduced fruit set, or deformed fruits. Fungal infections, in particular, can affect the

blossoms and developing
fruits.

6. **Genetic Factors:**

   - The plant's genetic makeup
     plays a significant role in its
     ability to produce fruits.
     Some varieties may be more
     resilient to environmental
     stressors, diseases, or pests.

7. **Nutrient Deficiencies:**

   - Inadequate levels of
     essential nutrients, such as
     nitrogen, phosphorus, or
     potassium, can limit the
     plant's reproductive
     capacity. Regular soil
     testing and appropriate
     fertilization are crucial for
     addressing nutrient
     deficiencies.

Management Practices:

1. **Pruning and Training:**

- Incorrect pruning techniques or inadequate training of the plant can impact fruiting. Pruning should be carried out at the right time and in the right manner to promote healthy growth and fruit development.

2. **Fertilization Schedule:**

- Improper timing or quantity of fertilizers can disrupt the nutrient balance in the soil. A well-defined fertilization schedule based on the plant's growth stages is essential for optimizing fruit production.

3. **Disease and Pest Management:**

- Integrated pest management strategies and disease control measures should be implemented to minimize

fertilization can address
these issues.

9.3.3 Weather-Related Challenges:

1. **Frost Damage:**

   - Late spring frosts or early fall frosts can damage tender plants and disrupt the normal growth cycle. Protective measures such as frost blankets or selecting frost-resistant varieties can mitigate the impact.

2. **Excessive Heat or Drought:**

   - Prolonged periods of high temperatures or drought can stress plants, leading to reduced yields. Mulching, proper irrigation, and choosing drought-tolerant varieties are essential in such conditions.

9.3.4 Weeds and Competition:

1. **Weed Control:**

   - Weeds compete with crops for water, nutrients, and sunlight. Effective weed management through cultivation, mulching, or herbicides is crucial for maintaining plant health and optimizing yield.

9.3.5 Soil Health:

1. **Erosion and Soil Structure:**

   - Soil erosion and compaction can negatively impact root growth and nutrient availability. Implementing erosion control measures and promoting soil aeration are essential for maintaining optimal soil health.

addressing poor fruit production and other common problems requires a holistic approach that considers both environmental and management factors.

Regular monitoring, timely interventions, and the implementation of sustainable agricultural practices are key elements in fostering healthy and productive fruit-bearing plants.